# THE PERFECT BALANCE WORKBOOK

*A Journey to a Healthier You!*

## Pam Sherman

# CONTENTS

# INTRODUCTION

This is going to be a way to take care of yourself and your health. This workbook is for the woman who wants change. She wants to take the time to plan out her health and fitness dreams and goals. She wants to get her food and exercise habits on track. She wants to get to her very best self!

I want you to feel better in your own skin, to wake up knowing you are taking care of yourself and your health every single day!

This workbook will help you change behaviors and patterns that are holding you back from your healthiest self.  I want to help you get to the place where you feel amazing in your own skin. Where you feel awesome in your clothes and feel confident when you look in the mirror day in and day out.

Oftentimes, we struggle to make changes stick. We want a healthier life but fall back on what we know and old habits. Old habits got you to where you are right now. I want to empower you to make the needed changes to reach your goals.

In this workbook, you will focus on making small changes that will lead to BIG success in your health and wellness. Changing too many things at once will just lead to disaster.

This will also be your place to reflect, journal your gratitude, answer some tough questions as well as be honest with yourself.

I hear many women say they have tried everything to lose weight and get healthier - that nothing works!

Losing weight and getting healthier is not a fast process. There is no quick fix. You don't gain 10 pounds overnight, nor will you lose 10 pounds overnight.

This time, I do NOT want you to quit on yourself. I want you to take this commitment to yourself and your health seriously.

We only have one body to go through life. I want you to treat yourself like your health is the most precious commodity in the world–which it is.

Success is NOT an overnight process. It takes consistency day in and day out. I want you to **NEVER** lose sight of what you want to accomplish.

I also want you to keep in mind how you are going to do that. It's not glamorous or exciting. SUCCESS will happen with daily dedication and determination from YOU!

# YOUR WHY

Let's talk about the BIG reason you want to get healthier. It is not an easy answer. Your **WHY** needs to be HUGE. It needs to be important enough to you, so that you will want to make the necessary changes to be healthier.

Take the time to reflect on this. I want your WHY to be more than, "I want lose weight." What will you gain by losing weight? More energy? Live longer? Be able to play with your kids/grandkids? Why do you want to be healthier?

Once you have your WHY – write it on a sticky note and post it everywhere. In the kitchen, on your desk, in your car, in your bathroom. I want you to be crystal clear on the bigger picture.

WHY .... Why are you embarking on this journey?

How will your life change once you meet your goal(s)?

What can't you do right now that you want to because of your current health situation?

What is your biggest challenge in your health?

Write down an example of when you have had success in your life in regards to health/wellness...

How did you feel at this time?

What are the 5 things you do well daily? For example – drink enough water, eat veggies....

1.

2.


3.


4.


5.


What are 5 things you struggle with daily? For example – I don't get enough sleep, don't plan my meals, etc.

1.


2.


3.


4.

5.

Make a list of the foods you normally eat in a week:

Make a list of foods that are healthy that you enjoy eating:

We all generally know how we should eat for health, so describe what you think is lacking in your eating habits:

Write down what kind of exercise you typically get in a week:

Have you ever loved exercise? If so what do you love to do?

If not, what did you like to do as a kid? Oftentimes, we still like to move the way we did when we were young. By the way – YouTube is a great resource to find ways to move that are FUN!

How many hours of sleep do you get on average each night?

**Food Habits** to shoot for:
Eating lots of color each day (not including candy)! Loads of vegetables and fruit, protein (including meat, fish, eggs, legumes, tofu), healthy fats (avocados, nuts, nut butters, eggs, fish) and healthy carbs (sweet/regular potatoes, rice, beans, fruit, veggies).

Try to avoid fast or processed foods as much as possible and try to eat real food as much as possible.

**Sleep Habits** to shoot for:

Most of us need 6–8 hours of sleep a night. Some need more some need less. You should know what works for your body. Do what it takes to get your optimal amount most nights of the week!

**Exercise Habits** to shoot for:

We are meant to move our bodies every single day. Find what you like to do, and fit it into your week. The days you can't do it, walk everywhere. I know you will feel better after moving your body. You will never regret a workout!

Additional thoughts?

# YOUR GOALS

Let's talk about goals. What are yours? If not, get thinking about what you'd like to achieve both short and long term. Goals should be measurable, attainable, and realistic.

What are your goals? Write 3 short term goals achievable in 1-2 weeks.

1.

2.

3.

Now I want you to think of an action plan for each of your goals. For example: if your goal is to drink more water, your action plan would be to drink a glass with each cup of coffee/tea daily, as well as bring a water bottle with you in the car so you have water with you at all times.

Action Plan for:

Short-Term Goal #1:

Short-Term Goal #2:

Short-Term Goal #3:

Now write 3 long-term goals achievable in 8-12 weeks.

1.

2.

3.

Action plan for long-term Goals

Long-Term Goal #1:

Long-Term Goal #2:

Long-Term Goal #3:

What have been your biggest obstacles in reaching your goals in the past?

1.

2.

3.

4.

How do you think you will feel if you dedicate yourself working on your goals daily?

Write a short note to yourself here about how you will feel after you successfully reach one of your goals ...

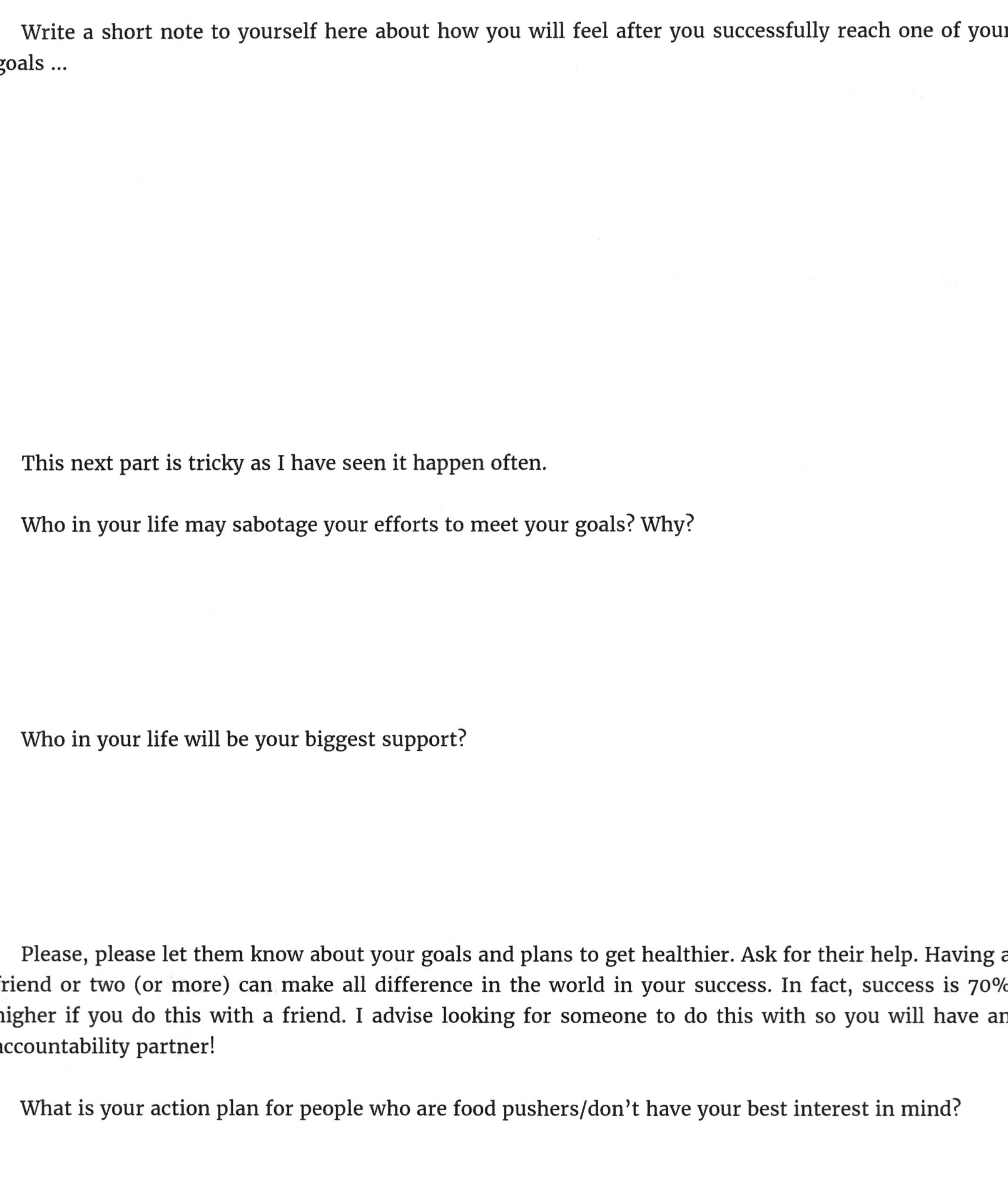

This next part is tricky as I have seen it happen often.

Who in your life may sabotage your efforts to meet your goals? Why?

Who in your life will be your biggest support?

Please, please let them know about your goals and plans to get healthier. Ask for their help. Having a friend or two (or more) can make all difference in the world in your success. In fact, success is 70% higher if you do this with a friend. I advise looking for someone to do this with so you will have an accountability partner!

What is your action plan for people who are food pushers/don't have your best interest in mind?

FYI- NO is a complete sentence when people are pushing food on you. Oftentimes saying NO to something is saying YES to yourself and your health!

What are the 5 things you are most thankful for?

1.

2.

3.

4.

5.

What do you LOVE the most about your body?

14

What do you find is your biggest struggle with your body?

Additional thoughts:

# YOUR PATTERNS & BEHAVIORS

What patterns do you have that you know you need to break? (A pattern is something you might do every day, or most days of the week, that you need to break.)

1.

2.

3.

What do you think the most important steps are going to be for you to feel great about yourself?

How can you incorporate these steps into your life?

Are you aware of behavior/s that may not be serving you right now? Ex: mindless eating, eating your feelings, eating when you're not hungry ... what are they?

How can you change or eliminate these in order to reach your goals?

If yes, are you ready to change these behaviors so you will feel better?

Do you have ideas on how you can change?

Do you currently put yourself on your daily calendar for food/exercise?

If not, why?

What do think has been holding you back from having the body that you want?

Are you ready to make changes, feel great about yourself and have a more positive outlook on your health and fitness?

Why now?

Please go back and re-read your answers (daily!) and know why it's important for you to stay committed to yourself.

Lastly – write a letter to your future self. Talk about what this journey meant to you and how you feel about yourself. Remember– YOU ARE WORTH THE TIME AND ENERGY IT TAKES – EVERY SINGLE DAY!

# YOUR FOOD JOURNAL

They say it takes 3 weeks to change! I want you to honestly and accurately journal every day for 21 days. This will show you patterns that are good. Patterns you need to change, patterns that don't serve you.

This journal is only for you. No one else will ever see it. Take the time daily to fill it out.

I KNOW in our super convenient and quick world, this is not quick or convenient.

BUT ... I also know that anything worth having takes work. In regards to your health, it will always take time to make changes for the better.

Your positive attitude and effort will make all the difference in you being successful on this journey or not. The choice is yours!

Now, let's get started ...

# DAY 1: DAILY FOOD JOURNAL

List 3 things you're grateful for today:

1.

2.

3.

First meal – list time and food:


How did you feel afterwards?


Second meal – list time and food:


How did you feel afterwards?


Third meal – list time and food:


How did you feel afterwards?


Snacks – list times and foods:


Overall, how do you think you did with your food today?


*Things to pay attention to: Are you really hungry? Are you tired? Bored? Lonely? Frustrated? Are you full after you eat? Are you planning your food or just grabbing and go?*

# DAY 2: DAILY FOOD JOURNAL

List 3 things you're grateful for today:

1.

2.

3.

First meal – list time and food:


How did you feel afterwards?


Second meal – list time and food:


How did you feel afterwards?


Third meal – list time and food:


How did you feel afterwards?


Snacks – list times and foods:


Overall, how do you think you did with your food today?


*Things to pay attention to: Are you really hungry? Are you tired? Bored? Lonely? Frustrated? Are you full after you eat? Are you planning your food or just grabbing and go?*

# DAY 3: DAILY FOOD JOURNAL

List 3 things you're grateful for today:

1.

2.

3.

First meal – list time and food:


How did you feel afterwards?


Second meal – list time and food:


How did you feel afterwards?


Third meal – list time and food:


How did you feel afterwards?


Snacks – list times and foods:


Overall, how do you think you did with your food today?


*Things to pay attention to: Are you really hungry? Are you tired? Bored? Lonely? Frustrated? Are you full after you eat? Are you planning your food or just grabbing and go?*

# DAY 4: DAILY FOOD JOURNAL

List 3 things you're grateful for today:

1.

2.

3.

First meal – list time and food:


How did you feel afterwards?


Second meal – list time and food:


How did you feel afterwards?


Third meal – list time and food:


How did you feel afterwards?


Snacks – list times and foods:


Overall, how do you think you did with your food today?


*Things to pay attention to: Are you really hungry? Are you tired? Bored? Lonely? Frustrated? Are you full after you eat? Are you planning your food or just grabbing and go?*

# DAY 5: DAILY FOOD JOURNAL

List 3 things you're grateful for today:

1.

2.

3.

First meal – list time and food:

    How did you feel afterwards?

Second meal – list time and food:

    How did you feel afterwards?

Third meal – list time and food:

    How did you feel afterwards?

Snacks – list times and foods:

Overall, how do you think you did with your food today?

*Things to pay attention to: Are you really hungry? Are you tired? Bored? Lonely? Frustrated? Are you full after you eat? Are you planning your food or just grabbing and go?*

# DAY 6: DAILY FOOD JOURNAL

List 3 things you're grateful for today:

1.

2.

3.

First meal – list time and food:


How did you feel afterwards?


Second meal – list time and food:


How did you feel afterwards?


Third meal – list time and food:


How did you feel afterwards?


Snacks – list times and foods:


Overall, how do you think you did with your food today?


*Things to pay attention to: Are you really hungry? Are you tired? Bored? Lonely? Frustrated? Are you full after you eat? Are you planning your food or just grabbing and go?*

# DAY 7: DAILY FOOD JOURNAL

List 3 things you're grateful for today:

1.

2.

3.

First meal – list time and food:


How did you feel afterwards?


Second meal – list time and food:


How did you feel afterwards?


Third meal – list time and food:


How did you feel afterwards?


Snacks – list times and foods:


Overall, how do you think you did with your food today?


*Things to pay attention to: Are you really hungry? Are you tired? Bored? Lonely? Frustrated? Are you full after you eat? Are you planning your food or just grabbing and go?*

# DAY 8: DAILY FOOD JOURNAL

List 3 things you're grateful for today:

1.

2.

3.

First meal – list time and food:


How did you feel afterwards?


Second meal – list time and food:


How did you feel afterwards?


Third meal – list time and food:


How did you feel afterwards?


Snacks – list times and foods:


Overall, how do you think you did with your food today?


*Things to pay attention to: Are you really hungry? Are you tired? Bored? Lonely? Frustrated? Are you full after you eat? Are you planning your food or just grabbing and go?*

# DAY 9: DAILY FOOD JOURNAL

List 3 things you're grateful for today:

1.

2.

3.

First meal – list time and food:

How did you feel afterwards?

Second meal – list time and food:

How did you feel afterwards?

Third meal – list time and food:

How did you feel afterwards?

Snacks – list times and foods:

Overall, how do you think you did with your food today?

*Things to pay attention to: Are you really hungry? Are you tired? Bored? Lonely? Frustrated? Are you full after you eat? Are you planning your food or just grabbing and go?*

# DAY 10: DAILY FOOD JOURNAL

List 3 things you're grateful for today:

1.

2.

3.

First meal – list time and food:


How did you feel afterwards?


Second meal – list time and food:


How did you feel afterwards?


Third meal – list time and food:


How did you feel afterwards?


Snacks – list times and foods:


Overall, how do you think you did with your food today?


*Things to pay attention to: Are you really hungry? Are you tired? Bored? Lonely? Frustrated? Are you full after you eat? Are you planning your food or just grabbing and go?*

# DAY 11: DAILY FOOD JOURNAL

List 3 things you're grateful for today:

1.

2.

3.

First meal – list time and food:


How did you feel afterwards?


Second meal – list time and food:


How did you feel afterwards?


Third meal – list time and food:


How did you feel afterwards?


Snacks – list times and foods:


Overall, how do you think you did with your food today?


*Things to pay attention to: Are you really hungry? Are you tired? Bored? Lonely? Frustrated? Are you full after you eat? Are you planning your food or just grabbing and go?*

# DAY 12: DAILY FOOD JOURNAL

List 3 things you're grateful for today:

1.

2.

3.

First meal – list time and food:


How did you feel afterwards?


Second meal – list time and food:


How did you feel afterwards?


Third meal – list time and food:


How did you feel afterwards?


Snacks – list times and foods:


Overall, how do you think you did with your food today?


*Things to pay attention to: Are you really hungry? Are you tired? Bored? Lonely? Frustrated? Are you full after you eat? Are you planning your food or just grabbing and go?*

# DAY 13: DAILY FOOD JOURNAL

List 3 things you're grateful for today:

1.

2.

3.

First meal – list time and food:


How did you feel afterwards?


Second meal – list time and food:


How did you feel afterwards?


Third meal – list time and food:


How did you feel afterwards?


Snacks – list times and foods:


Overall, how do you think you did with your food today?


*Things to pay attention to: Are you really hungry? Are you tired? Bored? Lonely? Frustrated? Are you full after you eat? Are you planning your food or just grabbing and go?*

# DAY 14: DAILY FOOD JOURNAL

List 3 things you're grateful for today:

1.

2.

3.

First meal – list time and food:


How did you feel afterwards?


Second meal – list time and food:


How did you feel afterwards?


Third meal – list time and food:


How did you feel afterwards?


Snacks – list times and foods:


Overall, how do you think you did with your food today?


*Things to pay attention to: Are you really hungry? Are you tired? Bored? Lonely? Frustrated? Are you full after you eat? Are you planning your food or just grabbing and go?*

# DAY 15: DAILY FOOD JOURNAL

List 3 things you're grateful for today:

1.

2.

3.

First meal – list time and food:


How did you feel afterwards?


Second meal – list time and food:


How did you feel afterwards?


Third meal – list time and food:


How did you feel afterwards?


Snacks – list times and foods:


Overall, how do you think you did with your food today?


*Things to pay attention to: Are you really hungry? Are you tired? Bored? Lonely? Frustrated? Are you full after you eat? Are you planning your food or just grabbing and go?*

# DAY 16: DAILY FOOD JOURNAL

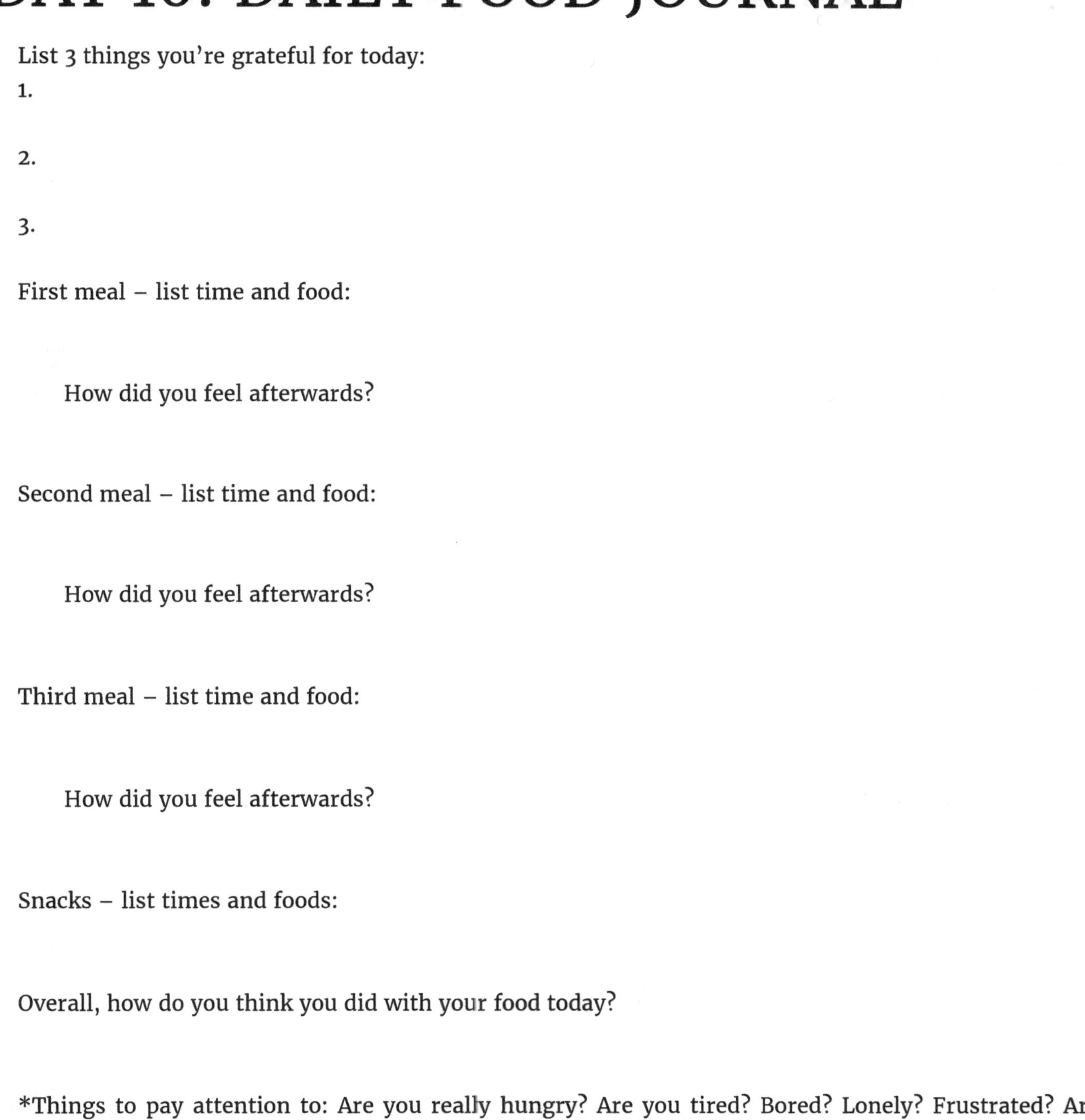

List 3 things you're grateful for today:

1.

2.

3.

First meal – list time and food:

How did you feel afterwards?

Second meal – list time and food:

How did you feel afterwards?

Third meal – list time and food:

How did you feel afterwards?

Snacks – list times and foods:

Overall, how do you think you did with your food today?

*Things to pay attention to: Are you really hungry? Are you tired? Bored? Lonely? Frustrated? Are you full after you eat? Are you planning your food or just grabbing and go?*

# DAY 17: DAILY FOOD JOURNAL

List 3 things you're grateful for today:

1.

2.

3.

First meal – list time and food:

How did you feel afterwards?

Second meal – list time and food:

How did you feel afterwards?

Third meal – list time and food:

How did you feel afterwards?

Snacks – list times and foods:

Overall, how do you think you did with your food today?

*Things to pay attention to: Are you really hungry? Are you tired? Bored? Lonely? Frustrated? Are you full after you eat? Are you planning your food or just grabbing and go?*

# DAY 18: DAILY FOOD JOURNAL

List 3 things you're grateful for today:

1.

2.

3.

First meal – list time and food:


How did you feel afterwards?


Second meal – list time and food:


How did you feel afterwards?


Third meal – list time and food:


How did you feel afterwards?


Snacks – list times and foods:


Overall, how do you think you did with your food today?


*Things to pay attention to: Are you really hungry? Are you tired? Bored? Lonely? Frustrated? Are you full after you eat? Are you planning your food or just grabbing and go?*

# DAY 19: DAILY FOOD JOURNAL

List 3 things you're grateful for today:

1.

2.

3.

First meal – list time and food:

How did you feel afterwards?

Second meal – list time and food:

How did you feel afterwards?

Third meal – list time and food:

How did you feel afterwards?

Snacks – list times and foods:

Overall, how do you think you did with your food today?

*Things to pay attention to: Are you really hungry? Are you tired? Bored? Lonely? Frustrated? Are you full after you eat? Are you planning your food or just grabbing and go?*

# DAY 20: DAILY FOOD JOURNAL

List 3 things you're grateful for today:

1.

2.

3.

First meal – list time and food:

How did you feel afterwards?

Second meal – list time and food:

How did you feel afterwards?

Third meal – list time and food:

How did you feel afterwards?

Snacks – list times and foods:

Overall, how do you think you did with your food today?

*Things to pay attention to: Are you really hungry? Are you tired? Bored? Lonely? Frustrated? Are you full after you eat? Are you planning your food or just grabbing and go?*

# DAY 21: DAILY FOOD JOURNAL

List 3 things you're grateful for today:

1.

2.

3.

First meal – list time and food:


How did you feel afterwards?


Second meal – list time and food:


How did you feel afterwards?


Third meal – list time and food:


How did you feel afterwards?


Snacks – list times and foods:


Overall, how do you think you did with your food today?


*Things to pay attention to: Are you really hungry? Are you tired? Bored? Lonely? Frustrated? Are you full after you eat? Are you planning your food or just grabbing and go?*

NOTES

# ADDITIONAL RESOURCES

Subscribe for weekly inspiration, follow us on Facebook, and discover more great resources at:

## www.theperfectbalance.guru

**Programs by Pam Sherman:**
SEXY in 60 Days! (**S**elf-confident, **E**nough, **X**traordinary **Y**ou!)

Are you tired of how you look and feel? SEXY in 60 Days is for you! It works body and mind to get your SEXY back. This is not a quick fix. It's a way to get your body/health back on track forever! Schedule your free consultation at theperfectbalance.guru/sexy

**More books by Pam Sherman – available on Amazon:**
- 21 Days to a Leaner & Healthier You – Small, Easy Changes to Help You Look and Feel Better
- Your Health is Your Wealth – 60 Inspirations for Fitness, Motivation and Resilience
- Healthy Living Guide – No-Nonsense Wisdom for Better Health
- Rules for Weight Loss – No-Nonsense Wisdom for Long-Term Success
- How to Avoid the Freshman 15 – No-Nonsense Wisdom for Health & Fitness in College
- Nutrition for Athletes – No-Nonsense Wisdom for Peak Performance

NOTES